YOUR KNOWLEDGE HAS VALUE

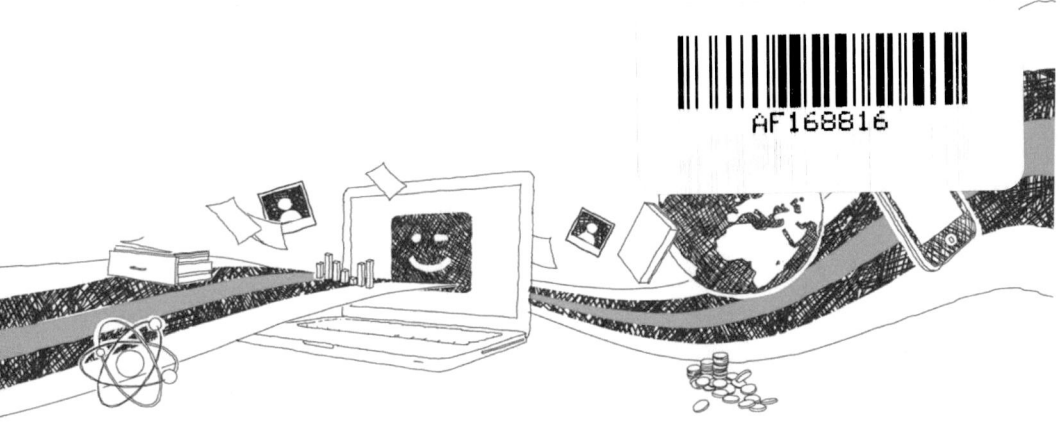

- We will publish your bachelor's and master's thesis, essays and papers

- Your own eBook and book - sold worldwide in all relevant shops

- Earn money with each sale

Upload your text at www.GRIN.com
and publish for free

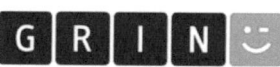

Bibliographic information published by the German National Library:

The German National Library lists this publication in the National Bibliography; detailed bibliographic data are available on the Internet at http://dnb.dnb.de .

This book is copyright material and must not be copied, reproduced, transferred, distributed, leased, licensed or publicly performed or used in any way except as specifically permitted in writing by the publishers, as allowed under the terms and conditions under which it was purchased or as strictly permitted by applicable copyright law. Any unauthorized distribution or use of this text may be a direct infringement of the author s and publisher s rights and those responsible may be liable in law accordingly.

Imprint:

Copyright © 2018 GRIN Verlag
Print and binding: Books on Demand GmbH, Norderstedt Germany
ISBN: 9783668725669

This book at GRIN:

https://www.grin.com/document/428632

Leonard Kahungu

Healthcare Systems in the US and UK. A Comparison

GRIN Verlag

GRIN - Your knowledge has value

Since its foundation in 1998, GRIN has specialized in publishing academic texts by students, college teachers and other academics as e-book and printed book. The website www.grin.com is an ideal platform for presenting term papers, final papers, scientific essays, dissertations and specialist books.

Visit us on the internet:

http://www.grin.com/

http://www.facebook.com/grincom

http://www.twitter.com/grin_com

STRUCTURED COMPARATIVE CASE STUDY REPORT
By (LKW)

Table of Contents

Introduction 2
A. Country Description 2
B. Health System 3
   1. Brief History of Health System 3
   2. Description of Current Health System 4
      2.1 Facilities 4
      2.2 Workforce in Health System 5
      2.3 Public/Private Health Services 5
      2.4 Cost of Healthcare 5
      2.5 Quality of Healthcare 6
      2.6 Access 6
   3. Evaluation of Healthcare System 7
      3.1 Cost 7
      3.2 Quality 8
      3.3 Access 8
   4. Emerging Health Issues 9
C. Conclusion 12
Recommendations 12
References 13

Introduction

Health care delivery systems and financing structures are some of the most popular across the globe when it comes to the wellbeing of the human race. The resultant popularity is influenced by the significance of universal healthcare and the efficiency levels attributed to healthcare delivery, financing, and accessibility, among other factors (Simonet, 2015). All countries are inherently predisposed to have unique healthcare financing and delivery systems due to assorted issues such as political history, culture, economic, and demographic factors. In particular, health care in the United Kingdom and the United States has been at the centre of political, social, and cultural debate in the past few years.

A. Country Description

On the one hand, the United States of America (USA) commonly abbreviated as the US, gained its independence as a country and subsequently created and ratified its initial constitution along with the national government between 1776 and 1789. In 1789, the nationalist movements in the US repealed the Articles of Confederation in attempts to authority and mandate of the federal government's authority in defence along with taxation with the Constitution of the USA, which is still in operational till to date (Zinn, 2015). The US is made up of 50 states and a number of territories extending into the Pacific Ocean, with a size of about 9.8 million squared kilometres. The large size is accompanied by geographic variety with an assorted types of climates across the country. It is prone to hurricanes and some of the worst known tornadoes in the world.

The US population is estimated to be at 325,719,178 people in 2017, which has quadrupled from an average of 76 million at the beginning of the 20th century. The White Americans make about 73.1% of the total population, while the African Americans are considered as the largest minority group (Zinn, 2015). Others large racial minority groups are grouped as Hispanic and Latino Americans. It is estimated that about 82% of the American population live in urban areas and suburbs. The US macroeconomic aspects are considered as capitalist mixed economy, which is enhanced by vast natural resources and extraordinary productivity, with a GDP of $16.8 trillion (Zinn, 2015). It is estimated that about 12.7% of the total population live in poverty. The transport and energy sector are highly developed, while the basic literacy is estimated to be 99%, and the education index is pegged at 0.97.

On the other hand, the United Kingdom of Great Britain and Ireland, simply referred to as the United Kingdom (UK), or Britain begun in 1707 with a political unity and collaboration of England and Scotland monarchies, while the Kingdom of Ireland was later added 1800. The modern Britain is made up of England, Scotland, Wales and the Northern Ireland, which are largely made up of islands, while its size is estimated to be 248,532 square kilometres. The UK is considered as the sixth largest economy in the globe with a GDP of $2.619 trillion, as of 2016. It has the strongest GDP across the European region (Floud et al., 2014). As of 2011, the UK population was estimated to be 63,182,000, with England recording the highest population density. The literacy level is relatively high and it is estimated to be 99% at the age of fifteen years, which is attributed to the universal public education that was established in 1890. The UK population is dominated by the White Britons, with the immigrants making up to 13% of the total population (Floud et al., 2014). It is estimated that 6.5%, an equivalent of about 3.9 million people live in what is described as persistent income poverty.

B. Health System

1. Brief History of Health System

The US healthcare system is considered as a hybrid system as it is offered my numerous organisation with unique characteristics. It is estimated that about 58% of the community hospitals are non-profit, 21% are privatised while 21% are publicly funded by the government (Osborn et al., 2016). The US is among the few member states of the OECD that fail to include healthcare as a basic human right and also does not guarantee availability of access to healthcare. The hybrid nature of the US health care system implies that different entities, private and public provider healthcare services in the country (Malhotra et al., 2015). In particular, the primary providers include health care facilities, healthcare personnel, along with medical products. The largest financier is the federal government in collaboration with the state and local authorities through special programs such as Veterans Health Administration, Medicaid, the Children's Health Insurance Program along with Medicare (Shaheen et al., 2018). A significant portion of the American citizens who fail to qualify for the special programs enrol to private insurance programs with a range of merits and demerits. Health indicators are described as quantifiable features in a community or civilization that are used as supporting evidence characterising the wellbeing of a population. These indicators are established by the Healthy People 2020 objectives, which reflect the primary health concerns in the US (Case and Deaton, 2015). These factors include access to healthcare, mental health, injury and violence, environmental quality, physical activity, immunisation, responsible sexual behaviour, tobacco use and substance abuse along with overweight and obesity (Lorenzoni et al., 2014). Notably, the Healthy People framework is subject to modifications after every ten years based on the health status of the US population.

The UK healthcare system is a devolved function with Scotland, Northern Ireland, Wales and England having unique systems that are publicly funded and accountable to different governments within their respective jurisdictions. Voluntary provisions and private sector make a small portion of the UK healthcare system (Devaux, 2015). The National Health Service (NHS) is a common body in the UK that oversees the provision of healthcare services for free or subsidised costs to all the legal UK citizens. The UK government is the largest financial provider of healthcare services through taxation, with a record of 98.8% funding. However, specific policies are different in the four kingdoms of the Great Britain (Buescher et al., 2014). The publicly funded system is based on the notion that universal healthcare system is the right of all Britons living in the UK. The NHS was first launched in 1948, with the subsequent years seeing numerous amendments and modifications to suit the population needs. The primary health indicators are based on the NHS Health Outcome Framework, which is centred on health life expectancy between communities, improved health expectancy and reduced differences in life expectancy (Squires, 2011). Noticeably, the mortality and morbidity rates have significantly improved in the UK and the US in the 21st century, but preventable and chronic diseases remain a significant threat to the healthy populations in both nations.

2. Description of Current Health System

2.1 Facilities

The ownership of the US healthcare system is privatised, but the federal, state, and local governments have their own facilities. The US lacks a countrywide government owned health facilities that are open for the general public consumption, yet the local government owns a number of medical facilities that are opened for the general public (Jakovljevic, 2016). The healthcare systems in the UK is largely owned by devolved governments but healthcare in England is provided by the NHS. The largest NHS hospital in England is known as the Norfolk and Norwich University Hospital (Gilbert et al., 2015). Healthcare in Northern

Ireland is provided through the Health and Social Care in Northern Ireland, while in Scotland and Wales by NHS. The private hospital forms a very small niche with a 2% in England.

2.2 Workforce in Health System

Most physicians are trained under the US medical education system, whereby all practitioners are required to acquire medical license within the state jurisdictional mandate. An increase of US spending on healthcare has triggered an increase of the workforce in the sector, in which one in every eight Americans work in the healthcare related field, accounting for an average of 10% of the country's workforce (Bekelman et al., 2016). Since the UK healthcare system is largely funded by the central and devolved governments, the workforce is accountable to the NHS. It is estimated that NHS employs more than 1.3 million workers in the healthcare sector, making it the largest employer in the UK (Malhotra et al., 2015). In both instances, an increased demand for social health workers has soared due to the growing population of the senior citizens due to favourable socioeconomic factors.

2.3 Public/Private Health Services

As previously observed in the report, the US healthcare system is predominately made up of the private services providers, including the insurers and facilities and practitioners. The federal government funds healthcare facilities and the entire industry through special programs and arrangements, which makes the healthcare system a hybrid industry due to the presence of public, private, and not-for-profit collaborative efforts (Himmelstein et al., 2014). On the contrary, the UK healthcare system is largely universal, whereby healthcare is seen as an entitlement and a human right. However, there exists private healthcare providers, which forms a significantly small portion in the healthcare industry.

2.4 Cost of Healthcare

The US healthcare is considered as the most expensive system compared to other industrialised or OECD countries. The cost has significantly escalated from at the beginning of the 21st century but it is believed to have slowed as of 2011. For each dollar spent towards the healthcare services, 31% is consumed by the hospital care, which includes diagnostic, outpatient and hospital spending per visit and discharge (Squires and Anderson, 2015). Others include 21% which directed to physicians/clinical services, and 10% to pharmaceutical products, 4% to dental care, 6% is absorbed by the nursing homes, 3% to home health care settings, 3% for complementary retail products, 3% to the government's public health initiatives. 7% of each dollar spent is directed to administrative costs, 7% to investment programs while 6% is consumed by other professions (Filardo et al., 2016). The publicly funded healthcare in the UK accounts for more than 79.5% of the total spending £ 147.1 billion. Specific expenditure differs between the major kingdoms with England recording the highest spending.

2.5 Quality of Healthcare

Compared to the UK, the quality of the US healthcare system is largely considered inefficient. This is due to heavy annual spending, the absence of universal healthcare, and poor accessibility in the midst of escalating healthcare costs (Ryan et al., 2016). However, the UK healthcare system is considered above average compared to other countries due to increased heavy spending and poor health indicators affecting the country (Himmelstein et al., 2014).

2.6 Access

The physician and hospital supply along with spending in the US entails 2.43 practicing physician per 1,000 people, while the acute care hospital beds per 1000 population 2.7. The average length of stay for acute care is 5.5 days, while the hospital discharge per 1000 population is 130 and the total health spending in 2008 was $897 (Squires, 2011). The UK total health spending was $368 in 2008. The practicing physicians per 1000 population was 2.61 and the acute hospital beds per 1,000 was 2.7. the average of length of stay for acute care 7.1 and the hospital discharges per 1000 was 136.

Exhibit 4. Supply and Utilization of Doctors and Hospitals in Select OECD Countries, 2008

	Physician Supply and Use		Hospital Supply, Use, and Spending		
	Practicing physicians per 1,000 pop.	Doctor consultations per capita	Acute care hospital beds per 1,000 pop.	Average length of stay for acute care (days)	Hospital discharges per 1,000 pop.
Australia	2.97[a]	6.4	3.5[b]	5.9[b]	163[a]
Canada	—[f]	5.7[a]	2.7[a]	7.5[a]	84[a]
Denmark	3.42[a]	8.9	3.0	—[f]	159
France	—[f]	6.9	3.5	5.2	264
Germany	3.56	7.8	5.7	7.6	232
Netherlands	—[f]	5.9	2.9	5.9	113
New Zealand	2.46	4.3[a]	2.2	—[f]	140
Norway	4.01	—[f]	2.5	4.8	172
Sweden	3.58[b]	2.9	—[f]	4.5[a]	165[a]
Switzerland	3.82	4.0[a]	3.3	7.7	169
United Kingdom	2.61	5.9	2.7	7.1	136
United States	2.43	4.0[a]	2.7[a]	5.5	130[b]
OECD median	3.00	6.4	3.3	6.0	161

a 2007
b 2006
f Data not available
Source: OECD Health Data 2010 (Oct. 2010)

Figure 1: Source (Squires, 2011)

3. Evaluation of Healthcare System

3.1 Cost

According to the World Health Organisation, the US healthcare expenditure was about 17.8% of the total GDP in 2016 translates to $3.2 trillion. Per capita expenditure in 2014 was established as $8,054. It was projected that this would increase to 19% by 2017 while the healthcare per capita cost to $9,990 (Squires, 2011). The expenditure in 2016 indicates that the national health cost was over 3.3 trillion. Health spending by major source of funds indicates that the government through Medicare and Medicaid spend 20% and 17%, respectively, which translate to $672.1 billion in 2016 and $565.5 billion, respectively. Private health insurance spent 34% of the total expenditure, which translates to $1.1 trillion in 2016. Lastly, the out-of-pocket expenditure was 11% or 352.5 billion in the same year. In the United Kingdom, the NHS was 98.8% from the national insurance along with taxation (Squires, 2011). Particularly, the UK spends about 9.8% of its GDP on the healthcare, which is equivalent to £138 billion annually. It is estimated that the NHS spends about £2009 per person throughout the UK. In England, the costs translate to £1,992 per person, Wales £1,998 per individual, while in Scotland and Northern Ireland £2,150 and £2,115 per person, respectively. The private sector funding has experienced a significant increase to 10% of the NHS total expenditure in 2015, which is equivalent to £9 billion (Squires, 2011).

3.2 Quality

Life expectancy, mortality rates, vaccinations and fertility rates play a central role in indicating the quality of the healthcare system in a country. Over the past few years, the life expectancy in the UK has slightly improved. A male born in the UK could live up to 79.2 years while a female could live up to 82.9 years if the mortality rates were to remain the same as of 2016. The mortality rate in the UK is estimated to be 9.4 deaths per 1000 population as of 2017. Nonetheless, these statistics are likely to differ when it comes to age and geographical distribution, with England recording the highest death rate compared to other kingdoms. The fertility rate has also improved over the past years as illustrated by the contemporary data. There are 11.6 live births recorded per 1000 population in the UK, as of 2016 (Simonet, 2015). On the other hand, the US mortality rate was reported to be 8.4 per 1000 people in 2016. Life expectancy at birth is estimated to be 78.74 years as of 2015, cutting across population features. The fertility rates in the US is 62 live births per 1000 women as of 2016 (Squires, 2011). Malnutrition, especially for children under the age of five years was measured last in 2014 and was established to be 25.20. Lastly, it is estimated that about 0.7% of the children living in the US did not receive any vaccination in 2013.

3.3 Access

Healthcare in the UK is considered an entitlement as well as a basic human life. This is the primary reason there is a universal healthcare system, which guarantees accessibility and equitability in the UK. Thus, most people are eligible for the universal healthcare services in the UK population. Nonetheless, the immigrants living in the UK are largely left out of the universal healthcare plans due to eligibility concerns (Osborn et al., 2016). It is estimated that over 12% of the Britons are covered under the voluntary health insurance also known as private medical insurance schemes. On the contrary, the US healthcare system is largely on the private hands, which means that its distribution primarily depends on the profitability metrics. As a consequence, a significant portion of unemployed individuals fail to secure sustainable healthcare coverage plans (Malhotra et al., 2015). Most people in the rural areas are also not in a position to access timely and quality care services due to the physical absence of healthcare facilities. This is attributed to commercialisation causes, since most healthcare facilities are concentrated on densely populated areas. The increasing cost of healthcare in the US also make such plans unsustainable (Shaheen et al., 2018). Moreover, healthcare disparities are some of the leading challenges facing the US. This is attributed to complex socioeconomic and political factors, such as racism and other forms of discrimination, which discourage minority groups from seeking the primary healthcare.

Exhibit 9. Hospital Admissions for Chronic Diseases and Diabetes Amputations in Select OECD Countries, 2007

	Hospital Admissions for Chronic Diseases per 100,000 Population, Age 15 and Older					Diabetes lower extremity amputations per 100,000 population, age 15 and older
	Asthma	Chronic obstructive pulmonary disease	Congestive heart failure	Hypertension	Diabetes acute complications	
Canada	18	190	146	15	23	11
Denmark	43	320	165	85	20	21
France	43	79	276	—*	—*	13
Germany	21	184	352	213	14	—*
Netherlands	26ᵇ	154ᵇ	171ᵇ,ᵈ	19ᵇ	8ᵇ	11ᵇ
New Zealand	73	308	206	16	1	12
Norway	42	243	188	70	20	11
Sweden	25	192	289	61	19	12
Switzerland	32ᵃ	100ᵃ	155ᵃ	55ᵃ	12ᵃ	16ᵃ
United Kingdom	76	236	117	11	32	9
United States	120ᵃ,ᶜ	203ᵃ,ᶜ	441ᵃ,ᶜ	49ᵃ,ᶜ	57ᵃ,ᶜ	36ᵃ,ᶜ
Median (countries shown)	42	192	188	52	19.5	12

Age-sex standardized rates. Data not available for Australia.
ᵃ 2006
ᵇ 2005
ᶜ U.S. does not fully exclude day cases

Figure 2: Source (Squires, 2011)

4. Emerging Health Issues

Being among the industrialized countries, both the UK and the US are significantly affected by health related conditions. This is attributed to increased sedentary lifestyles in developed countries. Particularly, it is estimated that as of 2012 one on every four adults were diagnosed with one or more chronic conditions in the US (Case and Deaton, 2015). It was also established that seven out of ten causes of deaths in 2014 were linked to chronic conditions. Among the chronic diseases, cancer and the heart disease accounts for over 46% of all deaths in the US. Obesity was isolated as the major health concern in the American population. Statistics indicates that about 36% of all adults in the US had obesity between 2011 and 2014. Arthritis is considered as the leading cause of disability in the US while diabetes was the main cause of kidney failure, and the amputation of the lower limbs along with other complications related to diabetes (Lorenzoni et al., 2014). These trends are primarily attributed to the presence of multiple players in the healthcare industry, which increase the cost of seeking primary healthcare services. This is evident in marginalised communities, whose prevalence of preventable conditions and diseases are higher than the majority populations. Lack of long-term and affordable health coverage in the majority of the US population is another factor influencing the contemporary trends of healthcare (Devaux, 2015). In the midst of escalating healthcare costs and unaffordable comprehensive healthcare coverage plans, most American citizens are fail to seek timely medical care, which is paramount in improving intervention outcomes.

Exhibit 11. Rates of In-Hospital Case-Fatality Within 30 Days of Admission in Select OECD Countries

	In-Hospital Case-Fatality Within 30 Days of Admission per 100 Patients, 2007		
	Acute myocardial infarction	Hemorrhagic stroke	Ischemic stroke
Canada	4.2	23.2	7.6
Denmark	2.9	16.7	3.1
Netherlands	6.6ᵇ	25.2ᵇ	5.6ᵇ
New Zealand	3.3	23.8	6.3
Norway	3.2	13.7	3.3
Sweden	2.9	12.8	3.9
United Kingdom	6.3	26.3	9.0
United States	5.1ᵃ	25.5ᵃ	4.2ᵃ
Median (countries shown)	3.8	23.5	4.9

Note: Figures do not account for death that occurs outside of the hospital, possibly influencing the ranking for countries, such as the U.S., that have shorter lengths of stay. Medicare data is available on 30-day mortality in the U.S., but this is not currently available from private insurers.
Age-sex standardized rates (%). No data available for Australia, France, Germany, or Switzerland.
ᵃ 2006
ᵇ 2005
Source: OECD Health Care Quality Indicators Data 2009

Figure 3: Source (Squires, 2011)

Correspondingly, arthritis has also been identified as the leading cause of disability in the UK, in which about 8 to 10 million Britons suffer from Arthritis. There are about 1.3 million individuals living with diabetes in England and the figure are expected to increase upwards in the coming years. Diabetes has is also attributed to an increase of coronary heart diseases along with stroke. It is estimated that about 110,000 suffer their first stroke in every year (Jakovljevic, 2016). Moreover, stroke is identified as the leading cause of death in the United Kingdom, among other countries. Most trending health concerns in the UK are similar to those observed in the American population, except for unique particulars that have slight variations. These trends are also mirrored in industrialised countries, which are largely attributed to sedentary lifestyles in these populations. However, inefficiencies in the UK's healthcare system are associated with the monopolisation of the healthcare system (Buescher et al., 2014). There are calls for the privatisation of the healthcare in the UK in attempts to increase its efficiency and reduce various inefficiencies associated with the entire system. It is believed that privatisation would increase the care delivery capacity and also eliminate various inefficiencies currently witnessed in the care system.

Exhibit 8. Supply, Use, and Price of Diagnostic Imaging in Select OECD Countries

	MRI Machines			CT Scanners	
	Devices per million pop., 2008	Exams per 100,000 pop., 2008	MRI scan and imaging fees, 2009[g]	Devices per million pop., 2008	Exams per 100,000 pop., 2008
Australia	5.6	21[d]	—[f]	56.0[b,e]	94[d]
Canada	6.7[a]	42	$824	12.7[a]	122
Denmark	—[f]	38	—[f]	21.5	84
France	—[f]	49	$436	—[f]	130
Germany	—[f]	—[f]	$839	—[f]	—[f]
Netherlands	10.4	39	$567	10.3	60
New Zealand	9.6	—[f]	—[f]	12.4	—[f]
Switzerland	—[f]	—[f]	—[f]	32.0	—[f]
United Kingdom	6.9	—[f]	$179	10.2	—[f]
United States	25.9[a]	91[a]	$1,200	34.3[a]	228[a]
Median (countries shown)	8.3	40	$696	17.1	108

Note: Data on CT scanners and MRI units do not include those outside hospitals in Germany and only for a small number in France. For the United Kingdom, the data refer only to scanners in the public sector. For Australia, the number of MRI units includes only those eligible for reimbursement under Medicare; the universal public health system; in 1999, 60% of total MRI units were eligible for Medicare reimbursement. Also for Australia and France, data for CT and MRI exams refer only to utilization by out-patients and private in-patients (excluding those in public hospitals). Data not available for Norway or Sweden.
[a] 2007
[b] 2006
[d] Difference in methodology
[e] Estimate
[f] Data not available
[g] Source: International Federation of Health Plans, 2009 Comparative Price Report.
Source: OECD Health Data 2010 (Oct. 2010), unless otherwise specified

Figure 4: Source (Squires, 2011)

C. Conclusion

Evidently, the UK and the US healthcare systems share numerous characteristics, which are also common in other industrialised countries (Bekelman et al., 2016). These similarities are primarily based on the economic status along with the socio-political features in these countries. However, there are unique differences between the two nations. For instance, whereas the US healthcare system is a mixture of private and public organisations, the UK care system is largely funded by the government (Gilbert et al., 2015). The commercial orientation of the healthcare system is the US has stimulated an escalation of the healthcare costs, increasing the accessibility disparities throughout the country. On the other hand, the public funding of the UK's healthcare system has contributed to its inefficiencies due to wastages and alleged misappropriations.

Recommendations

Apparently, both the US and UK healthcare system are characterised by multiple defects that require socioeconomic and political interventions. The major recommendation for the US healthcare system is centred at eliminating healthcare disparities by addressing affordability issues. An increase of the private organisations has increased administrative costs along with the commercialisation of essential healthcare necessities (Malhotra et al., 2015). This has partly led to the increase of healthcare costs, which reduces the accessibility and affordability. Therefore, the commercialisation aspect in the US healthcare system should be monitored to arrest the escalating healthcare costs. On the other hand, major inefficiencies are attributed to public funding, with marginalised contributions from the private sector. This calls for the increase privatisation of the healthcare system, in attempts to enhance or supplement the capacity of the healthcare provision and address the existing issues.

References

Bekelman, J.E., Halpern, S.D., Blankart, C.R., Bynum, J.P., Cohen, J., Fowler, R., Kaasa, S., Kwietniewski, L., Melberg, H.O., Onwuteaka-Philipsen, B. and Oosterveld-Vlug, M., 2016. Comparison of site of death, health care utilization, and hospital expenditures for patients dying with cancer in 7 developed countries. *Jama*, *315*(3), pp.272-283.

Buescher, A.V., Cidav, Z., Knapp, M. and Mandell, D.S., 2014. Costs of autism spectrum disorders in the United Kingdom and the United States. *JAMA pediatrics*, *168*(8), pp.721-728.

Case, A. and Deaton, A., 2015. Rising morbidity and mortality in midlife among white non-Hispanic Americans in the 21st century. *Proceedings of the National Academy of Sciences*, *112*(49), pp.15078-15083.

Devaux, M., 2015. Income-related inequalities and inequities in health care services utilisation in 18 selected OECD countries. *The European Journal of Health Economics*, *16*(1), pp.21-33.

Gilbert, F., Tucker, L., Gillan, M., Willsher, P., Cooke, J., Duncan, K., Michell, M., Dobson, H., Lim, Y., Purushothaman, H. and Strudley, C., 2015. The TOMMY trial: a comparison of TOMosynthesis with digital MammographY in the UK NHS Breast Screening Programme-a multicentre retrospective reading study comparing the diagnostic performance of digital breast tomosynthesis and digital mammography with digital mammography alone.

Filardo, G., da Graca, B., Sass, D.M., Pollock, B.D., Smith, E.B. and Martinez, M.A.M., 2016. Trends and comparison of female first authorship in high impact medical journals: observational study (1994-2014). *bmj*, *352*, p.i847.

Floud, R., Humphries, J. and Johnson, P. eds., 2014. *The Cambridge Economic History of Modern Britain: Volume 1, Industrialisation, 1700–1870*. Cambridge University Press.

Himmelstein, D.U., Jun, M., Busse, R., Chevreul, K., Geissler, A., Jeurissen, P., Thomson, S., Vinet, M.A. and Woolhandler, S., 2014. A comparison of hospital administrative costs in eight nations: US costs exceed all others by far. *Health Affairs*, *33*(9), pp.1586-1594.

Jakovljevic, M.M., 2016. Comparison of historical medical spending patterns among the BRICS and G7. *Journal of medical economics*, *19*(1), pp.70-76.

Lorenzoni, L., Belloni, A. and Sassi, F., 2014. Health-care expenditure and health policy in the USA versus other high-spending OECD countries. *The Lancet*, *384*(9937), pp.83-92.

Malhotra, A., Maughan, D., Ansell, J., Lehman, R., Henderson, A., Gray, M., Stephenson, T. and Bailey, S., 2015. Choosing Wisely in the UK: the Academy of Medical Royal Colleges' initiative to reduce the harms of too much medicine. *Bmj*, *350*, p.h2308.

Ryan, A.M., Krinsky, S., Kontopantelis, E. and Doran, T., 2016. Long-term evidence for the effect of pay-for-performance in primary care on mortality in the UK: a population study. *The Lancet*, *388*(10041), pp.268-274.

Simonet, D., 2015. The new public management theory in the British health care system: a critical review. *Administration & Society*, *47*(7), pp.802-826.

Shaheen, A.A., Somayaji, R., Myers, R. and Mody, C.H., 2018. Epidemiology and trends of cryptococcosis in the United States from 2000 to 2007: A population-based study. *International journal of STD & AIDS*, *29*(5), pp.453-460.

Squires, D. and Anderson, C., 2015. US health care from a global perspective: spending, use of services, prices, and health in 13 countries. *The Commonwealth Fund*, *15*, pp.1-16.

Squires, D.A., 2011. The US health system in perspective: a comparison of twelve industrialized nations. *Issue Brief (Commonwealth Fund)*, *16*, pp.1-14.

Osborn, R., Squires, D., Doty, M.M., Sarnak, D.O. and Schneider, E.C., 2016. In new survey of eleven countries, US adults still struggle with access to and affordability of health care. *Health Affairs*, *35*(12), pp.2327-2336.

Zinn, H., 2015. *A people's history of the United States: 1492-present*. Routledge.

YOUR KNOWLEDGE HAS VALUE

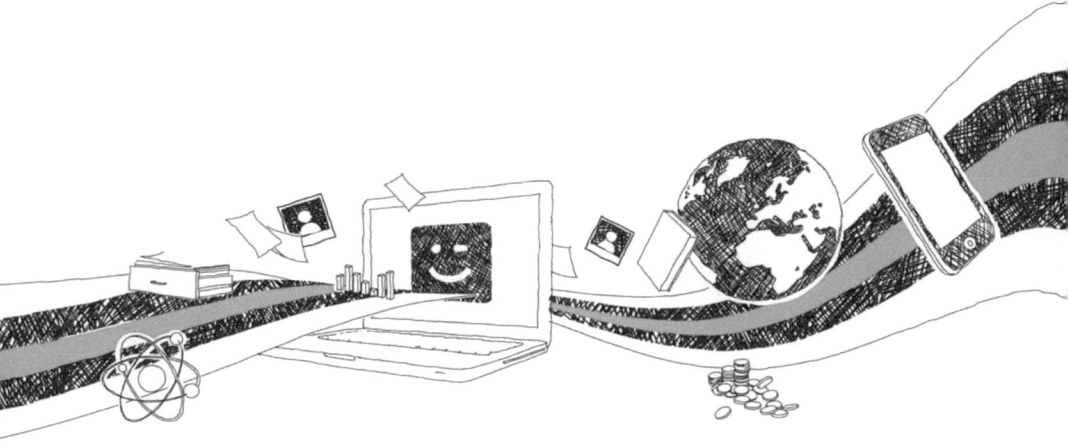

- We will publish your bachelor's and master's thesis, essays and papers

- Your own eBook and book - sold worldwide in all relevant shops

- Earn money with each sale

Upload your text at www.GRIN.com and publish for free

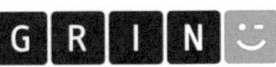